Hard Body Pain and Massage Therapy Solutions

HOW STRESS CREATES HARD BODIES IN PAIN

Martin Kunsman

I wish to express my gratitude to Jim Gabriel, Ann Pauley, Dr. Rudy Scarfalloto, Elizabeth Sundby, Patricia Kilpatrick, and Dr. Linda Westman.

TABLE OF CONTENTS

INTRODUCTION

This book is for educational purposes only. It is not intended to contradict, or replace the advice of your physician.

This book is a compilation of three books. It is a bit repetitive if you read all three parts. Part One is a quick question and answer session for those who want to skim the important points. Part 2 is an in-depth look at the same topics as Part 1. Part 3 is in the form of a lecture or talk on the same material with more of an emphasis on massage therapy. This book is for those who want to live a healthy pain free life without having to resort to pain pills and expensive surgeries. I also think the ideas in this book are important because the fitness centers and personal trainers seem to be focusing on making the body more tone, not less.

This book describes 5 revolutionary concepts about the musculo-skeletal system:
1. Stress creates hard bodies.
2. Hard bodies have more pain issues.
3. Hard bodies have more digestive issues.
4. A massage therapist can tell you if you are a soft body or a hard body.
5. Cardio exercise softens hard bodies.

Hopefully, in the near future, we will see softening the resting muscle tone as a popular fitness goal. There seems to be a bit of a disconnection between the people who are touching bodies and the people who are training them. Also, those who are helping with pain issues seem to be relying more on MRIs and X-rays rather than good old fashioned palpation or investigative touch. We can hope that one day in the future, all of the specialties of therapeutic massage, psychotherapy, fitness training, physical therapy and orthopedic surgery all come together in a unified system for helping those in pain.

Part One

HARD BODY PAIN AND

QUICK ANSWERS

Chapter 1

BODIES WITH THE LEAST PAIN

ARE OFTEN THE SOFTEST

Do you work on keeping your body healthy and pain free? Do you ever wonder what a healthy body looks like and feels like? From a musculoskeletal view, a healthy body looks and feels soft. The muscles are not hard when they are at rest. Muscles should be long with full range of motion. Muscles should be soft when they are at rest. I am a massage therapist and I am amazed at how many people have very hard, dense muscles. Even when they are at rest, the muscles feel hard. At rest, not flexing, their hand and forearm muscles will feel hard. At rest, not flexing, their upper trapezius muscles will feel hard. Moving throughout their body and palpating the muscles will yield the same sensation.....a hard dense body. Let's call these people Hard Bodies. **The more I talk to Hard Bodies, the more I become convinced that they have more pain conditions in their bodies than their opposites, the Soft Bodies.** We have so many syndromes these days that we should give this a name. Let's call it, "Hard Body Pain Syndrome." Not only do they usually have more pain but they will tell you about another thing they often have in common.....Stress.

With my experience feeling muscle tension or tone on hundreds of people and talking to them about their lifestyle, I have come to the conclusion that Soft Bodies have much less pain issues than Hard Bodies. Further, this condition can be reversed if they find a way to let go of the stress they are holding in their body.

Healthy muscles at rest are soft, pliable, and flexible. I should be able to sink my fingers into your muscles. If the muscles all over your body keep fingers from pressing into them with even moderate pressure, you are a Hard Body.

We are going to talk about how to soften the resting tone of the body. We are also going to talk about how to become more flexible. We are going to talk about therapeutic massage therapy. All of these topics are really about one thing…..**Creating Space**.

Creating space in the body can be thought of like a balloon that has space to expand. Hard bodies are like tight balloons. They barely budge when you press into them. There is no space. Soft bodies are like balloons that are less filled with air. When you press into them, there is plenty of room for you to press into them.

Flexible muscles are longer. They have more space. So, stretching and yoga can create more space.

Massage therapy can create some space.

Our Nervous System can create more space.

A chiropractic adjustment must create more space.

Surgery might create more space.

Keep this in mind while reading. Practitioners can create space but there are many things you can do on your own to create a soft, pliable, flexible body

Chapter 2

WHY ARE THE SOFTEST BODIES

MORE LIKELY TO BE FREE FROM PAIN?

Maybe it's because the softer muscles allow more room for the nerves and skeletal system to find their balance. Perhaps, the muscular and nervous system will make the shifts to keep us out of pain if they can. Maybe the skeletal system and the nerves have more room to move around the way they want to. A soft body is easier to work with as a massage therapist if I am trying to help them with pain issues. I just find the areas in their body where they are holding some tightness and try to release this area. A hard body is hard all over so the investigation is much more difficult.

Chapter 3

IS PAIN ALWAYS RELATED TO

RESTING MUSCLE TONE?

Pain conditions are not always related to muscle tone. Some pain is not caused by an imbalance of the musculoskeletal system. There could be many other factors. For instance, disease, burns, or straining a muscle. There are many pain conditions that are not related to the subject of this book.

Chapter 4

HOW DO HARD BODIES

BECOME HARD?

They seem to be the people living a stressful life and not releasing this stress but holding it in their bodies. They may have an imbalance in the parasympathetic and the sympathetic nervous system. (See Chapter 6.) Some diseases create hard bodies. I don't have much experience with people with these serious diseases.

Chapter 5

MANY HARD BODIES

HAVE DIGESTIVE ISSUES

It seems that all of the Hard Body people I talked to also had digestive issues.

This will make more sense after reading the next chapter. This may be due to an imbalance of the parasympathetic and sympathetic nervous system. (See next Chapter.)

Chapter 6

HOW MIGHT OUR NERVOUS

SYSTEM CREATE A HARD BODY?

Hard Bodies may be created from an imbalance of the nervous system, The following comes out of my course work at ASHA massage school.

The Nervous System consists of the nerves that branch out from the Central Nervous System and connect it to other parts of the body. The **Peripheral Nervous System** contains the **Somatic System** and the **Autonomic System.**

The **Somatic System** consists of motor neurons that are under voluntary control. Every time we decide to pour a glass of water or get up from a chair we are using these neurons that are under our voluntary control to move us around.

The **Autonomic System** consists of neurons that are under involuntary control. It works automatically without us directing it. **Through our lifestyles we can have a huge effect on this system.** It can be broken down into a side that speeds things up and readies our body for action and a side that slows things down and allows our body to recover and relax.

The side that speeds things up is called the **sympathetic division.** The side that slows things down is the **parasympathetic division.**

The **sympathetic** side is in charge of speeding things up and preparing our bodies for action when we are threatened. It is known as the "fight or flight"part of our nervous system. Our bodies have been designed from years and years of having to survive in the wild. Animals chasing us for food, etc... Whenever we are under attack our sympathetic nervous system readies our body for action. It does this by tensing our muscles slightly, speeding up our breathing, increasing our heart rate and stimulating our brains. The one area it slows things down is digestion. So it speeds everything up when we are in this "fight or flight" mode except digestion which it slows down. Now why do you think our body decreases digestion during this time? It is a way our body prioritizes during an emergency. When there is a threat our body does not want to use any precious energy on digestion, there will be time for that later.

The **parasympathetic** side slows everything down, **except digestion** which it speeds up. The parasympathetic system decreases muscle tone, slows down our breathing and heart rate. The threat is over and we don't need our bodies readied for fight or flight. When we are in fight or flight mode we don't have to be doing our digesting during this time, we may not be around if we don't instead direct that energy to our muscles and our breathing, etc... Once the threat is gone the parasympathetic side slows everything down and increases digestion which we now have time for.

What is happening in our fast paced society is the **sympathetic** system which is only supposed to kick in during emergencies is being stimulated way too much.

So our heartbeat gets up, our breathing, our muscle tone increases and our digestive system gets put on hold. This may create the Hard Body and the Hard Body Pain Syndrome. When it is finally time for our **parasympathetic** system to come and slow everything down again we aren't giving it enough time or the right atmosphere to calm everything down. The **parasympathetic** system gets bogged down with way too much work because the **sympathetic** system created all of this tension in our bodies. It's supposed to be a balancing act but the **sympathetic** "fight or flight" part of our nervous system has created havoc. Our bodies will get hard and create pain issues and digestion issues.

Chapter 7

HOW DO SOFT BODIES

BECOME SOFT?

Chapter 3 guessed at why Hard bodies are hard. Now let's guess at why Soft Bodies are Soft. Soft Bodies seem to be people who don't hold any stress in their bodies. They either live very peaceful, stress free lives or they just don't hold onto stress. Very often it is someone that might have a fast paced life but they have a way of releasing the stress. Many Soft Bodies do cardio exercise.

Chapter 8

RECOMMENDATIONS FOR

SOFTENING YOUR BODY

I recommend you do cardio exercise. Massage therapy can soften tight specific areas, and can have a slight effect in softening overall muscle tone.

Part One

Chapter 9

WHAT ABOUT FLEXIBILITY?

People with pain issues often have lost some of their flexibility in a certain joint. For instance, lower back pain often comes from tight, short quadricep muscles. Increasing Range of Motion of a joint is a way of creating more space in the body. Flexibility creates space the same way having soft muscles create space in the body. Hard Dense muscles are locked down and need more room to move around. Flexibility indicates longer, softer, healthier muscles.

Hard bodies are like bricks. They barely budge when you press into them. There is no space. Soft bodies are like rubber erasers. You can press into them and they have more flexibility.

Chapter 10

HOW TO BECOME MORE FLEXIBLE,

CREATE MORE SPACE

I recommend yoga to anyone who wants to increase their flexibility or increase their range of motion for particular joints. Some types also give you a good cardio workout.

Chapter 11

WHAT ABOUT INCREASING TONE THROUGH

STRENGTH TRAINING?

Is strength training and building muscle tone important? Aren't healthy muscles also strong? I prefer to put these questions off until once we fully understand full range of motion and muscles that are soft when they are at rest. **Strength training and building muscle tone should always be secondary to range of motion and overall softness of muscles when they are at rest.** If you have full range of motion and your muscles are soft when they are at rest, then, you may be in a position to build some strength in certain areas. Tone and strength training are not the focus of this book. This book is focused on range of motion and softening muscles when they are at rest.

Chapter 12

WHAT ABOUT A SOFT BODY

THAT HAS A PAIN PROBLEM?

It could be a pain condition totally unrelated to the muscle tone. Or, it could be that a particular area of muscles has become too hard. It is common for a softbody to have lower back pain because they do a lot of core strength training. Be careful of the strength training you do and don't continue if you think it is causing you pain. Listen to your body. Is there an area of tight muscles above or below where you are feeling pain? If your wrist hurts, are your forearms hard? Use this same question everywhere in the body. If your heel hurts, are your calves and achilles tendon too hard?

Also, you could be creating tight areas from your cardio training. Your overall muscle tone may make you a soft body but create tight IT bands, or glutes. Being a soft body makes this tight area easier to find and release with massage therapy.

Tight areas may be the result of an injury or a muscle strain. These areas need rest and light massage to let them heal.

It could be a bone or disk problem. This is outside the scope of what I do.

Tight areas can also be created by repetitive patterns such as sitting at a desk working on a computer or driving a car. Many people create tight areas by working Tennis players can create tight calves (soleus, gastroc), from all of that running on concrete. Massage therapist often have hard forearms. Restaurant managers and servers often have tight muscles in their feet and lower legs.

Some injuries create tight areas. You may strain a muscle in your knee and all of the muscles in the knee area stiffen to keep you from injuring the knee joint further.

Massage therapy can help release these tight areas. Also, consider a good flexibility program to increase the length of the tight muscles. It's all about creating space in the body. Creating softness where there is hardness. Creating space where things have gotten too bunched together.

Chapter 13

CONCLUSION

Softer Bodies often have less pain issues than harder, denser bodies. Massage therapist can tell us if we are Hard Bodies or Soft Bodies.

Hard bodies should do cardio exercise and get some relaxation type massage to help stimulate the relaxation part of their nervous system. Soft bodies should get massage therapy, for relaxation and also the type that releases specific tight areas. Yoga works well to soften those tight areas as well and helps with overall range of motion. Massage therapy should match the body. A person's exercise regimen should match what their body needs. Massage therapists and yoga instructors can help clients set personal workout goals.

Bodies should be monitored throughout a lifetime and assessed for any problem areas. Structure should be assessed and fitness plans and massage therapy work should be tailored towards improving structure.

Part Two

HARD BODY PAIN,

SOFT BODY BLISS

Chapter 1

SOFTER IS BETTER

I wrote the first edition of this book in 2006. At the time I predicted that muscle tone would be talked about more as more people got massage therapy. The massage therapy boom has definitely happened but I still don't hear much talk about resting muscle tone. I made this second edition easier to understand. I cut out most of the chapters on weight lifting, body structure, flexibility, and other topics. I realized that resting muscle tone should not be confused with all of those other topics. I'm trying to keep on topic and make this easier to understand this time around.

This book is for everyone. Anyone can benefit from the information described in this book. It is especially relevant for people who are currently experiencing pain on a daily basis. This is a more common occurrence than you may think. The little aches and pains that we carry with us from week to week are likely shared by our neighbors. Many of us have pain that progresses to the point where it is interrupting our sleep.

If you are someone who carries very little pain with them, this information will give you greater understanding as to why you are one of the fortunate ones. This understanding can help keep you healthy and you can share this message to your family and friends.

This book solves problems. The problem it solves is pain and digestion issues. I'm about to tell you how to get rid of a lot of pain so I want to define what kind of pain issues I'm talking about. Muscle pain and digestion issues are often related so we will say many digestion issues plus.....

Pain, tingling, numbness, weakness in the arms, hands, legs, or feet
  Back pain
  Headaches
  TMJ issues (pain, biting or grinding issues)
  Wrist pain (in the carpal tunnel region)
  Sciatic pain, numbness
  Upper back or neck pain
  Shoulder pain

This is a book that can give you insight into what a massage therapist can tell you about your body. Some of the best advice about the body is coming from people who touch them every day. The resting tone of the muscles is one of the biggest determinants in whether or not that person has pain. **The softer your body is, the less pain you will experience in your life**. That statement sets this book up as a revolution. It may become obvious to people who touch people and talk to them about pain but it is totally hidden from view by almost everyone else. This book describes what a healthy body feels like. There is a lot of confusion about what healthy muscle tone looks and feels like.

One of the most telling things about a person's body is the tone of their muscles. When I say tone of a muscle, I mean the resting muscle tone. If a person's resting muscle tone is too high or too hard, they will generally have pain issues with their bodies. Many people think, the firmer the muscles are, the better. This is not true. Firm hard muscle usually indicate pain or dysfunction for that individual. The tone is also an indicator that the person is holding stress in their bodies. A hard body is a good indicator that the person may be working too hard physically or mentally. It can also be an indicator of emotional stress for the individual. A massage therapist who puts their hands on people every day can give you a good idea if you are a hard body or a soft body. I used to think there was an in-between or a medium body. But the more people I work on the more I'm convinced that our bodies are either hard or soft. It's as if it is some kind of binary system where tone is being held or released. To measure how tone your muscles are, you need the right massage therapist to give you feedback. The number of people massage therapists have their hands on will give them a frame of reference to how your body feels relative to everyone else. If you are a hard body, this may explain many of the aches and pains you have been having lately. Looking around for that perfect pillow, or mattress is not really addressing the problem. The problem is the amount of tension that you are holding in your muscles. The way to reduce the hard feel in your muscles is to do aerobic training daily. I suggest yoga, jogging or biking. Also, try to reduce the amount of mental or emotional stress in your life. You may have to scale back on the hours you spend on work and try to schedule some quiet time for yourself.

This is a completely overlooked component of our health that needs to be addressed. With awareness we can then decide if the fast pace of our lives is worth the inevitable pain and discomfort that can affect our bodies. This will also influence how we work out. If our bodies are hard from the stress in our lives, the last thing we need, is to be lifting weights and making our bodies even harder. There is a lot of emphasis placed on the value of strengthening and toning our bodies. What is not always understood is how that strengthening will many times have the effect of making our muscles harder. I would like to see the emphasis placed on having healthy flexible, elastic muscles that have a nice soft tone to them when pressed.

The tone of our muscles should be one of the first things considered when we begin to have pain issues with our bodies. Unfortunately, I don't think the tone of muscles is ever even thought about as a source of the problem. Our medical profession rarely touches people or talks about muscle tone. It is an area that is sorely missing from U.S. traditional medical care.

This is such an obvious book for people who do massage therapy and who also talk to their clients that I am actually a little embarrassed to be writing it. I feel like it is a book on describing how the sky really looks blue. I knew that stress created a hard body within the first year of doing massage therapy. Why this book needs to be written is that so few people know that stress can create hard bodies that can create quite a bit of pain and dysfunction.

Why do so few people know this? I didn't know it until I became a massage therapist. I hugged people, I shook peoples' hands, I patted people on the back, but I never understood the connection between stress and hard bodies until I began massaging people every day. I've talked to many massage therapist who haven't noticed this connection yet. Perhaps they aren't talking to their clients and trying to connect the dots between lifestyle and body type.

I do not expect this book to be widely believed until a documentary is done on the subject. One lady asked me if there had been research done on the subject. I imagine research could be done but I think all that is really necessary is a documentary or "talk show" where someone could "read" the amount of stress a person is holding in their muscles. The obviousness of watching someone read a total strangers body is all of the research that most people will need to see.

When I am assessing a person's body, I am thinking of four things:
The overall tone of the person's muscles . . . softer is better.
The flexibility the person has in their hips, shoulders legs and arms...full range of motion is ideal.
Specific areas of tightness . . . everyone has at least a couple.
I am looking for symmetry in the persons structure....the hips, shoulders and spine

While reading this book, try to think about these four things and it will help you make sense of the book. The overall tone of a person's muscles is discussed in the first two chapters. Specific areas of tightness refer to where a person is holding more tension in certain muscles of their body. This may be due to just where they hold their mental/emotional stress. This may be the result of something they are doing over and over . . . building too much strength in those muscles creating tightness. A good example would be a mother who lifts her kids every day. Or, it may be the result of how they sit and where they sit every day. It may be due to something as simple as sitting at a computer every day.

Chapter 2

ARE YOU A HARD BODY

OR A SOFT BODY?

Pain is often the result of tight muscles that are tight because the person is holding stress there. To get rid of the pain, they need to soften that tight area in their body. The easiest way to soften muscles is through an aerobic workout such as yoga, running or biking. Another way to soften muscles is to reduce the stress from work and life in general.

Our view of a beautiful body is changing as we learn about what a healthy body looks like. The new beautiful and healthy body is the one that is most soft, rubbery and elastic. Someone who takes on a great deal of stress will often have hard and dense muscles. Since a hard body is generally thought of as a good thing in our society, they do not see this as a warning sign. When they begin to have pain, they will not connect the dots to their hard muscles.

Many individuals focus on how their body looks and plan their workout sessions accordingly. Many personal trainers also will focus on how certain parts of the body look. This tendency to focus on a look rather than feel leads many people down a path of a beautiful looking but not beautiful feeling body. Many things that look cool when you lift weights, bulk, definition and hardness, do not feel very good to the person living in those bodies. They are beautiful from a distance. A massage therapist will tell you many of those sculpted physiques are loaded with trigger points, joint dysfunction, posture and range of motion issues.

A healthy muscle will be soft to the touch. If you press with your fingers into a person's back, your finger should sink into the muscles. The more resistance to pressing, the harder their body is, and the more likely they will have pain issues such as back pain, shoulder pain, hip pain and headaches.

Imagine someone coming up to you and telling you your muscles are too hard. Would it make you laugh? Would you think the person crazy? Would you ignore them? This is the reaction most people have when I bring this topic up.

I have come up with a naming system that helps us to know our body type. I divide bodies into two categories.....Soft Bodies and Hard Bodies. These categories are not focused on a particular area of the body but the overall resting muscle tone of the entire body. It can be confusing because sometimes people have more tone in a certain area of their body. These names try to take those areas out of consideration and to try to get a feel for the overall bodies' resting muscle tone.

Hard Body

Hard bodies have very hard resting muscle tone. It's as if their muscles are never relaxing. Their bodies feel like countertops, hard and dense. These people are under an incredible amount of stress (usually from work stress or emotional stress). If you press on their backs, their legs, their arms, or their hands, they will be hard. These people usually have lower back pain. They may be experiencing headaches or tingling or numbness in their hands and feet. Their range of motion, or flexibility, is usually very bad. They may not be able to bend at the knees much past 90 degrees. They are many times but not always overweight. **An easy way of spotting a Hard Body is when you try to slide a few fingers underneath their shoulder blades, the muscles will not let you in even a quarter of an inch.**

Sometimes if I'm working on a Hard Body, I will tell them that they are holding a lot of stress in their muscles......if the conversation develops and they begin to ask questions about why they are holding stress, I will get into how the nervous system sets the tone of the muscles and I may casually ask them if they are having digestive issues....99 percent of the time they say yes....how did I know that a hard body usually has digestive issues?.....we will get to that in chapter four.

Recently, I gave a massage to a lady who was a Hard Body. She was very friendly and outgoing. She said a couple of things during the massage which told me she didn't really know how much stress she was holding in her body. She knew she was overweight, but she didn't know about the hardness of her body. Toward the end of the massage I said, "Your muscles are very hard as if you are holding a lot of tension . . . you must have a very stressful job." She seemed a little surprised that I could tell that about her. After a little pause, she decided it was safe to tell me the story. She had been a public school system teacher for more than 30 years. She was about to retire because she said she had given all she could to the public school systems. She went on to say how frustrated she was with the public school system she was working for. She said she had quit exercising three years ago because her workload had increased so much that she didn't have any energy for it. Many hard body types have stories about the how stressful their lives are. Two days ago another Hard Body told me the last two years had been filled with in-laws dying, parents dying, and her husband had been diagnosed with a serious illness. I have come to the conclusion that life is very hard for a lot of people and you can feel it in their bodies. It is important for them to know that this hard body can result in quite a few pain problems down the road....they usually are already experiencing pain issues.

Sometimes when I point out that they have hard, dense muscles and this is why they are experiencing various pains they say, "Oh yea, I should get more massage." As a massage therapist I will be able to soften their bodies some. For meaningful change, I think, they would have to do more cardio exercise.

Soft Body

Soft Bodies have the healthiest resting muscle tone. Their muscles have the softest feel when you press into them. However, they may have a few muscles that are tight and hard. Rarely do you find someone without any hard and tight muscles anywhere. This soft body has an overall muscle tone that is very soft. Their muscles are rubbery and elastic. It is possible to slide your fingers underneath their shoulder blades without the muscles completely you blocking you out. They usually have good or even great flexibility in their arms and legs. They may have stressful lives but they have found a way not to release the stress in their muscles. They are frequently people who do aerobic training during the week such as running or biking.

I was giving a massage the other day to this woman in her thirties that had the softest, healthiest body that you will ever feel. I told her 10 seconds into the massage that she was not holding much stress. She said, "well that's good." I asked her if she was a runner. Her back and neck soft muscles reminded me of a runner's body. She said "No, I just walk and do yoga." A few minutes later I found a few trigger points on some of her rotator cuff muscles. Almost everyone will have some tightness in this area, on top of the shoulder blades. As I continued to work on her, I continued to find nice, healthy muscles everywhere. She was holding a little tension in her glutes, but overall, very soft. I checked her flexibility of her legs while she was face down. Her flexibility was very good. She could bring her heel all the way to the glutes with no resistance at all from the quadriceps. It's common for soft bodies to be very flexible. Think about it, the muscles are long and pliable with no areas of tightness. They should be able to stretch a long way. Vice versa, hard bodies generally have very little flexibility(check out the chapter on flexibility.) Soft Bodies generally have no idea how different their bodies are from others. They have no idea how lucky and healthy they are. Hard Bodies don't know/care they are hard and the soft body people do not know/care they are soft. The soft body types do not recognize the value in having the soft muscle tone that they have. If you don't have pain, you may not know why you don't have it.

This is a new topic for many of us . . . since it is so new, you probably will not take my word for it. I encourage you to study this on your own. Begin trying to feel different body types of the people in your life. When you come across a soft body, interview them to try to discover why they are so relaxed. They may not be taking on much stress or they are taking it on but then finding ways to release it during the day.

When you find a hard body, interview them and find out why they are holding so much tension in their bodies. The stories will astound you. Ask them about pain issues they are having. The soft bodies will have fewer pain issues than hard bodies. They will also have fewer issues related to digestion.

You don't even have to put your hands on some people to know they have hard bodies. You can see it the way the skin is stretched too tight over the collarbones. You can see it in their upper traps, just above the shoulder blades... the muscles bulging, hard and tight. I have gotten to where I can feel it in a handshake.

I have added one more type that has been harder for me to categorize.....their muscles are hard or soft but there are little potmark/indentations you can see if you press into them. This must be some type of toxin, fat, or inflammation they are storing in their muscles. I think it's related to nutrition. Also, they are very sensitive to any pressure during a massage. Their muscles are sensitive to even medium pressure.

Chapter 3

LEARNING FROM EXTREME SOFTS

AND EXTREME HARDS

The musculoskeletal system works best when the muscles are kept soft and flexible. When the muscles get hard, the pain, tingling, numbness and weakness issues are likely to follow.

My first massage therapy job was working at a chiropractor's office. During the massage I would ask the client how they came to be getting chiropractic adjustments. They usually had a story about a day they woke up and could barely walk or bend over because they were in so much pain. The adjustments took them out of pain and allowed them to function again. After working there for about a year I began to notice how hard many of their bodies were. I wondered if the adjustments created space, took people out of pain, but didn't move them further along towards having a soft body. I wondered if the hard muscles had created the situation where they had all of that pain to begin with.

My next job in massage was working in high end hotels downtown. I began to make a connection between what people did for a living and the hardness of their body. I could predict how hard they were working. Many of the hotel clients were fast paced business people with a lot of responsibilities. I was able to learn from extremes. At the chiropractor's office I worked on people who were at the extreme end of hard bodies and at the hotel some of the people were at that same extreme. I found most hard bodies worked in a job with a lot of responsibility. However, sometimes they didn't work for a living but volunteered many places.

Many people don't want to talk during a massage and I usually don't talk much either, but, I would begin to ask a few questions at the end of their massage. It was like a game I started to play, predicting what their lives were like compared to what I felt in their bodies. It was very interesting because the body never lied. Sometimes I'd get upbeat stories from people whose body was telling me a harder story. I tended to believe the bodies.

The other extreme I learned from was the soft body extreme. Many people who are interested in their own health are beginning to get quite a few massages. So, about every tenth person would have these soft, healthy bodies. I would ask them what they did for a living or how they worked out. Many times the softest bodies were people who were runners. Runners hold much less tension in their muscles. Why do you think their muscle tone is nice and rubbery? I think they get out there and sweat and get their heart rate up and burn off some of the stress of the day. Sorry, that wasn't very technical, but I will get more technical later. For now, lets just think in common sense terms. If you hold a lot of stress in during the day, I will feel it in your body. On a personal note, whenever I run, bike, play tennis, or otherwise get my heart rate up, I have a calmer feeling throughout that day. Are my muscles softening?

What really encouraged me to keep studying this, was, if I ever had a room full of the same types. I have given quick sports massages to 50 runners before a 10k. Almost all Soft Bodies. I have given 50 chair massages at a meeting of managers from a large Fortune 500 company.... all Hard Bodies.

We are a country that values action, movement, responsibility. For many people quiet time or downtime seems like a waste of time. This quiet time is important because it allows us to restore balance to our bodies.

The other thing that this knowledge brings to the person is empowerment. If pain experts are always looking at deep structures but not talking about muscles, it gives the client the impression it is the result of an accident, natural phenomena, wear and tear, bad luck, old age, or genetics. The client never connects the dots between the hard body and the pain. And the hard body is something they can easily soften if they choose. It is difficult to see how emotions and work stress can cause a vertebra (bone) problem but easier to understand when you relate it to the muscles that hold that vertebra in place. How can stress affect a vertebra or a disk? But if you go one step back and ask what pulled that vertebra out of whack to begin with? What created the imbalance? . . . was it a muscle? . . . what makes muscles tight, short and prone to creating an imbalance? ......does a muscle really connect there? ......what can I do about it? .....does stretching help? These are questions that can lead the person back to personal choices. This throws the responsibility back to the person in pain. It is more difficult to tell a client it is their lifestyle that is creating the pain, but it is more empowering for them. Many times the best technology is touch and knowledge. The knowledge comes naturally to a massage therapist who is actively trying to determine how much tension the person is holding in their body. Hard bodies are not very happy bodies. You will begin to have pain issues with a hard body. Nerves must pass through muscle and if these muscles are too hard the nerve gets squished. You may get tingling and numbness in the hands and feet. This is very common. One of the first areas to get tight or hard on people is their neck muscles. All of the nerves that are on the way to the hand must pass through this neck region near the collarbone. This can result in tingling or numbness in the hands that almost all hard body types may experience. This condition is found in many people. It's easy to understand because all you have to think about are nerves being squished by a muscle that is too hard, similar to a water hose that loses pressure when you step on it. Do an internet search on thoracic outlet syndrome and learn all about it.

Headaches are commonly caused by tight muscles. This concept is more involved than the nerve compression problem but not that difficult to understand. Many massage schools are teaching something called Neuromuscular Therapy or Trigger Point Therapy.

Neuromuscular Therapy (NMT) is based on the fact that muscles refer pain into neighboring muscles. A headache might be caused by trigger points that are in neighboring muscles such as those around the shoulder blades. Trigger points can easily be identified, when you press into the muscle it may cause a twitch, an ache or pain in a totally different muscle. NMT can help many people with pain issues. Many times I work on people in an area just under their shoulder blade and it helps them with headaches or TMJ issues. Muscles refer pain and the location of pain may be a foot away from the muscles that are causing the pain. This relates to hard bodies because if your muscle gets hard it has a tendency to be full of trigger points. So it is a double threat, it can impinge a nerve or a joint or it can refer pain. Muscles are important! I love MRIs and X-RAYS, but therapists who touch people every day and understand the science behind it are just as valuable in educating you about pain.

There are so many things that can feel bad in a hard body that it is hard to list them all but I will give you an idea of some of them.

Hard Body Issues:

Pain, tingling, numbness, weakness in the arms, hands, legs, or feet.
Back pain
Headaches
TMJ issues (pain, biting or grinding issues)
Wrist pain (in the carpal tunnel region)
Sciatic pain, numbness
Upper back or neck pain
Shoulder pain

There is also a condition that goes along with this hard body: Issues with digestion.

Chapter 4

THE NERVOUS SYSTEM MAKES

YOU HARDER OR SOFTER

How does the body turn stress into a hard muscle? Have you ever gotten a little tense and felt tightening in your jaw muscles? That is a good example of how you body is reacting all over. To understand what is happening with our bodies under stress, we have to look at the nervous system.

The Nervous System consists of the nerves that branch out from the Central Nervous System and connect it to other parts of the body. The Peripheral Nervous System contains the Somatic System and the Autonomic System.

The Somatic System consists of motor neurons that are under voluntary control. Every time we decide to pour a glass of water or get up from a chair we are using these neurons that are under our voluntary control to move us around. Simple right? Now lets talk about the Autonomic System.

The Autonomic System is thought of as consisting of neurons that are under involuntary control. In other words, it works automatically, without us directing it. However, through our lifestyle, we can have a huge effect on this system. This system is made up of a side that speeds things up and readies our body for action, and a side that slows things down, and allows our body to recover and relax. The side that speeds things up is called the sympathetic division. The side that slows things down is the parasympathetic division.

The sympathetic side is in charge of speeding things up and preparing our bodies for action when we are threatened. It is known as the "fight or flight" part of our nervous system. Our bodies have been designed from years and years of having to survive in the wild. Whenever we are under attack, our sympathetic nervous system readies our body for action. It does this by tensing our muscles slightly (so we can run or fight,) speeding up our breathing, increasing our heart rate and stimulating our brains. In this mode our digestion system will slow down. So it speeds everything up when we are in this "fight or flight" mode except digestion which it slows down. Now why do you think our body decreases digestion during this time? It is a way our body prioritizes during an emergency. When there is a threat our body does not want to use any precious energy on digestion... there will be time for that later.

The parasympathetic side slows everything down. Well almost everything, except digestion which it speeds up. The parasympathetic system decreases muscle tone, slows down our breathing and heart rate. The threat is over and we don't need our bodies readied for fight or flight. When we are in fight or flight mode we don't have to be doing our digesting during this time, we may not be around if we don't instead direct that energy to our muscles and our breathing. Once the threat is gone, the parasympathetic side slows everything down and increases digestion which we now have time for.

What is happening in our fast paced society is the sympathetic system which is only supposed to kick in during emergencies is being stimulated way too much.

Our heartbeat gets up, our breathing, our muscle tone increases and our digestive system get put on hold. When it is finally time for our parasympathetic system to come and slow everything down again we aren't giving it enough time or the right atmosphere to calm everything down. The parasympathetic system gets bogged down with way too much work because the sympathetic system created all of this tension in our bodies. You see how it works, it's supposed to be a balancing act but the sympathetic "fight or flight" part of our nervous system has created havoc. Our bodies will get hard and create the pain issues mentioned above and our digestion system will begin to have issues as well. The sympathetic system shuts down the digestive system until a later time. Our body's digestive system will not be working very well. Generally, the harder the body, the more likely they are to have digestive issues.

What will happen shortly is people will begin to understand what healthy bodies feel like. There is a lot of emphasis on fat when I think the emphasis will switch to muscle tone. The words we use to describe the body will change. People might not say they want to tone up their muscles. Being hard will not be ideal. A pliable, rubbery, elastic body will now be seen as the pinnacle of physical and mental health.

Chapter 5

HOW TO SOFTEN YOUR MUSCLES

The softest bodies tend to be runners. I can spot a runner on my massage table in about four seconds because their muscles are elastic, rubbery, and pliable.

Some aerobic exercise will soften overall muscle tone but create tight or hard muscles in specific areas. For instance, swimming may create tight areas in the shoulder area while decreasing overall resting muscle tone throughout the body.

Look at the medicine aisle in a grocery store next time you are there. You will find several rows of pain medication. There will be a couple rows of things for upset stomach and constipation. The majority of the rest is for colds and allergies. If we focus on softening our bodies, the pain aisle will be needed much less. It's just masking symptoms not curing the problem.

The stomach pills for indigestion and constipation will be needed less as well. That leaves the cold medications. This is a bit off topic, but, I want to tell you about how I keep from getting colds. I used to get three or four colds a year. I used to think that it was normal. A few years ago I began getting eight hours of sleep a night and trying not to push myself too hard during the day. I never get colds anymore. It was totally a matter of rebuilding my immune system with rest. I think of colds like a headache, you don't want to think of them as normal or natural but rather something to learn from ..... what is my body trying to tell me.....am I pushing too hard? For me it is usually a signal to slow down and relax.

It seems that our mental and emotional states have a big influence on the muscle tone of our body. This can be offset somewhat by the exercise we get during the week. It's important that we do the right kind of exercise for our bodies. There are a lot of people with hard bodies that are thinking of going to the gym to start an exercise program of weight training(resistance training). From a soft body standpoint their time would be better spent doing an aerobic workout.

There might be devices in every home someday that measure resting muscle tone. There may be devices that measure all kind of health related numbers including resting muscle tone.

For most people I see the value in Yoga, and aerobic training. You also want to think about the environment you are working out in.

I went in a sporting goods store to see what products they offered in their fitness section. Most of the packages talked about toning up, firming up, etc . . . I think all of this marketing is taking us away from the truth. Keep looking, feeling and asking questions and I think you will see the benefit of keeping your body soft.

Chapter 6

CONCLUSION

I would like the general public to know what massage therapists are learning. I would like the yoga people to talk to the weight lifting people. It's as if no one is talking to each other. I think that massage therapists have a lot to share because they put their hands on people every day. My first real massage was at one of those massage school student clinics. During the massage I asked the therapist who was still in massage school what he thought. And he asked, "what do you mean?" I said, "well you put your hands on people every day I thought you might be able to tell me about my body." He didn't quite know how to respond but he said something like, "it feels like you are keeping yourself in shape." After giving hundreds of massages I don't think I have ever heard that question. Many people think massage therapists just rub. I don't think this is true of all a massage therapist, but a lot of them are feeling and noticing and comparing. And they say that the palpation skills increase over time. A therapist will be able to feel more the longer they work at the skill. That's kind of cool isn't it? So ask your therapist what they think. Ask them if they do assessments. Try to identify tight areas of your body and try to get them to soften. If you are lifting weights, make sure you are getting regular assessments to determine if you are developing trigger points, tight areas or decreasing your range of motion. Try to do yoga to build strength and flexibility. Many books have too much information to be interesting or useful. I hope that isn't the case with this book. Many times, we think only we have these little aches and pains but many people have them. I would like to summarize some of the themes we have been talking about.

First, a soft body is healthier than a hard body, from a musculoskeletal view.

Many people with pain or dysfunction have hard bodies.

Many soft body types will also have areas where they have pain. Their pain usually comes from a group of hard muscles in their body......perhaps coming from some type of workout they are doing or some kind of repetitive motion where they are building too much strength in an area. For instance, picking up a child or a dog, doing crunches, doing pushups, lifting weights, or swimming(which is hard on the shoulder muscles), etc...

A good way to soften your body is to do an aerobic exercise such as running, biking, life cycle, or yoga.

Keep the muscles flexible and strong by doing yoga.

Another good way to soften your body is to learn how to adopt a more relaxed way of life.

Another good way to soften your body is to create some relaxing time during the day.

Get massage and body assessments often.

Learn about nutrition.

Thank you for allowing me to work with you. Good luck on your adventure into living a pain free life.

Part Three

NEUROMUSCULAR MASSAGE

THERAPY TEACHING

Chapter 1

BACKGROUND

I want to begin this talk today with a little history about where I've been the last decade and how this might help you. I've been somewhat obsessed with pain. A lot of you are here because you have some kind of pain issue. Let me tell you how I got into Neuromuscular Massage Therapy. About 10 years ago I decided to go to massage school. Mainly because I was looking for something to go along with my tennis teaching career. My aunt had been a reflexologist and massage therapist as far back as the 1970s. I was always attracted to what she did. She seemed to be excited about studying the body. She always took seminars and learned as much as she could about healthy eating and living.

She would have loved to see all of the Whole Foods and Yoga Studios that have sprung up as more and more people have become part of this health revolution. It's not coming from the healthcare industry by the way. It's coming from a grassroots movement where people have begun to take responsibility for their health.

So, I wanted to be a massage therapist. I will never forget my first interview at the massage school I went to in Atlanta, Georgia. The director said in effect, "We are helping people with pain issues that are not being resolved with traditional healthcare.... We are fulfilling a need." This was Jim Gabriel. He and his wife had been teaching Neuromuscular Massage Therapy to Atlanta students since the 80s. Now, I'm all about doing things first or better, so, he was telling me just what I needed to hear. He had put together the finest, most passionate group of teachers that I had ever seen. Jim had the dream that we would all go out, rent space in a doctors office and do talks like this to recruit clients. This is why I'm here tonight, and it's why you're here.

The job I got out of massage school was working for chiropractors. The next job I had, which I had for 4 years, was working as a massage therapist for the high end hotels in Atlanta. I got my hands on a lot of people. Everyone was new each week. I would talk to them sometimes. I tried to put together what they talked about with their body. I sometimes guessed how they lived or what they were doing with their bodies. It was like detective work. The bodies held a mystery. Why do some bodies look and feel like this, while others look and feel like that? The massage school director, Mr. Gabriel was right about the need for serious massage. I always started each massage by asking if they had any pain issues they needed help with. Practically every person did. You think only you have a little pain issue you struggle with, but it in reality, everyone has a pain issue. It seemed strange doing this clinical type work in a hotel setting but that's where I found myself.

I was drawn to body assessment. Two years into that job I began writing a book based on what I had learned from the hotel work. The title of the book is, "Hard Body Pain, Soft Body Bliss." It was an account of the things I had observed with all of these bodies. All of these bodies' stories. One of the things that surprised me the most was that people who had a lot of stress in their lives had hard, dense muscles. I had never heard this before. Usually, the term, "hard body" was used as an analogy for someone who was a fitness fanatic, in shape. The fitness industry, I should say, weightlifting industry of the time, had created this perception that hard muscles were a good thing. Well, I was finding out, in my detective work, that they weren't a good thing. Hard muscles were usually an indication of someone with too much stress in their lives and also an indicator of pain. In my experience, softer was better. Why was no one talking about this? It is one thing for the public's perception about something to be a little off. But, to be exactly opposite.....this bothered me.

In massage school we talked more about specific tight areas known as trigger points. Or, we talked about how lifestyle could cause some muscles to become short and affect posture. What I was noticing was an overall muscle tightness that affected the whole body. You could feel it when you shook the person's hand. They were either a hard body or a soft body.

Chapter 2

WHAT HEALTHY LOOKS

AND FEELS LIKE

If hard is what not healthy feels like, what does healthy feel like? What does healthy look and feel like? It feels soft first of all. The muscles are not hard but supple. They may have some tight muscles in certain areas but not everywhere you touch. Next, the range of motion of all of the joints can be assessed. Not all soft bodies have perfect range of motion. However, it is usually at least in the middle range. Hard bodies usually have very little range of motion. Another thing I've noticed is that some people store toxins, perhaps fat, in their muscles. I will see many small circles under the skin when I press into the muscle. This person with this body type is very sensitive to touch. They can only handle a very gentle massage. This may be related to the liver needing help ridding the body of fats, so I've heard. I have them myself around the hip joint.

There are soft bodies, hard bodies, those with range of motion issues and those with toxins/fat in their muscles. Then, there are those with structural issues, such as a curve in their spine or hips that are not balanced. The hips can be imbalanced on two different planes. Looking at them from the front when the person is standing. Or, looking at a hip that might be higher when they are face down on the table. Those are the basic types I look for. The soft bodies usually have some areas of tightness somewhere if you look for them.

Chapter 3

VISUAL CUES OF A BALANCED

STRUCTURE AND POSTURE

The normal curve of a spine will bend forward at the lumbar region, bend back at the thoracics and bend forward again at the cervical spine. All of these curves are necessary because they give the spine the ability to flex like a shock absorber when we walk, jump or run. The spine is like a tree and the curves at our base will influence our upper curves. If the lumbar spine becomes too flexed forward the thoracic spine will compensate by bending too far back. Likewise, if the lumbar spine gets too flattened out, the thoracic region will also lose some of it's curve. Our spine is like a tree. The top curves are influenced by the curves below. Lets examine a neutral proper posture.

Neutral Posture

If you were standing in a neutral posture and a plumb line (a line directed straight down towards gravity) was hung from the top of the head to the ground, the line would pass approximately:

- Through the middle of the ear
- Through the middle of the shoulder joint
- Through the greater trochanter of the hip
- Just in front of the middle of the knee
- Just in front of the middle of the ankle joints

The above can be checked by a side view of the body. The body can also be examined for any imbalances when examined from the front. Is one shoulder higher than the other? Is one hip higher?

Also, the curve of the spine can be checked for any side bending or scoliosis.

Chapter 4

RANGE OF MOTION ISSUES

AFFECTING HIPS AND POSTURE

This expression ROM, range of motion, is a simple concept. It's how far you can move a joint, the arm or leg or other body part through a range of motion. For instance, if you are lying face down how far can you, bending at the knee, bring your foot to your glutes? Now this is just a classic example. If you are at the 90 degrees point then you probably have back pain. Ideally, you can bring your heel somewhat close to your glutes. This range is showing how long or flexible your quadricep muscles are. The longer they are the further your ROM on this exercise. If you understand this, you can understand every other muscle group. Why is ROM important? Because it visually shows you where the short and tight muscles are in the body.

First, lets talk about short and tight quadricep muscles. The visual we talked about a minute ago was how close the heel will come to the glutes. That's the visual. These muscles can get so tight that the hips actually tilt forward. This can affect the curve of the spine. The spine comes off the hips. So if the hips are tilted forward the spine comes off at too strong and angle. The lower or lumbar spine can come off at too strong an angle, the upper spine curves in the thoracics to compensate and the cervical spine compensates as well. Tight quadriceps can cause a lot of problems in the curve of the spine. A knowledge of anatomy helps in understanding ROM issues. We can draw pictures of the bones and see how the muscles pull them as they get tight.

Chapter 5

TIGHT PSOAS AFFECTING POSTURE

An often overlooked muscle which can affect structure or posture is the psoas iliacus muscle. It attaches at the lumbar spine and inserts at the lesser trochanter of the femur. When this muscle gets too tight it can create too much bend in the lumbar spine. Or it can limit the normal curve and cause a flattening of the lumbar spine. Understanding how these core muscles affect structure is key to understanding how to live a pain free life.

Chapter 6

RANGE OF MOTION

AFFECTING SHOULDERS

Another common thing I visually I see on the therapy table is ROM issues with the shoulders. Sometimes the pec muscles get tight and pull the shoulder joint forward. People in this case need to stretch the front of their bodies out. They need massage therapy and yoga to regain flexible, long, pliable pec muscles. Another thing I always check is the length of the latissimus dorsi muscle. This can affect the ROM of the shoulder joint as well.

Chapter 7

HARD BODY PAIN

The last two chapters talked about the muscle groups that affected structure. Tight quads can be seen by how they change the persons structure and posture. This next body type can be seen but it is easy to be felt. These are people who have hard dense muscles. You feel the tightness everywhere in their body. Once you have practice you can feel it in their handshake. Hard dense muscles are often the result of stress. When I feel a hard body, I ask them about their lives and they are usually holding onto a lot of stress for some reason. Their nerves and joints are encased in hard bodies that are like bricks or stones. No wonder they have so many problems with pain. The nerves must pass through these muscles. If the muscles are too hard it can begin to affect the nerves, which pass on a signal of pain, tingling or numbness..

To understand hard bodies you need to understand how our nervous system works.

This next part is from my book, "Hard Body Pain, Soft Body Bliss."

"How does the body turn stress into a hard muscle? Have you ever gotten a little tense and felt tightening in your jaw muscles? That is a good example of how you body is reacting all over. To understand what is happening with our bodies under stress, we have to look at the nervous system.

The nervous system consists of two main parts: The central nervous system (CNS) and the peripheral nervous system (PNS). The CNS contains the brain and the spinal cord. The PNS consists mainly of nerves that connect the CNS to every other part of the body. The peripheral nervous system contains the Somatic System and the Autonomic System. The Somatic System consists of motor neurons that are under voluntary control. Every time we decide to pour a glass of water or get up from a chair we are using these neurons that are under our voluntary control to move us around. Now lets talk about the Autonomic System.

This system doesn't get much attention because it is thought of as consisting of neurons that are under involuntary control. In other words, it works automatically without us directing it. However, through our lifestyles we can have a huge effect on this system. This system is broken down into a side that speeds things up and readies our body for action and a side that slows things down and allows our body to recover and relax. The side that speeds things up is called the sympathetic division. The side that slows things down is the parasympathetic division.

The sympathetic side is in charge of speeding things up and preparing our bodies for action when we are threatened. It is known as the "fight or flight" part of our nervous system. Our bodies have been designed from years and years of having to survive in the wild. Whenever we are under attack, our sympathetic nervous system readies our body for action. It does this by tensing our muscles slightly (so we can run or fight), speeding up our breathing, increasing our heart rate and stimulating our brains. In this mode, our digestion system will slow down. It speeds everything up when we are in this "fight or flight" mode except digestion which it slows down. Now why do you think our body decreases digestion during this time? It is a way our body prioritizes during an emergency. When there is a threat our body does not want to use any precious energy on digestion, there will be time for that later.

The parasympathetic side slows everything down. Except digestion, which it speeds up. The parasympathetic system decreases muscle tone, slows down our breathing and heart rate. What is happening in our fast paced society is the sympathetic system which is only supposed to kick in during emergencies is being stimulated too much.

Our heartbeat goes up, our breathing rate increases, our muscle tone increases and our digestive system gets put on hold. When it is finally time for our parasympathetic system to come and slow everything down again we aren't giving it enough time or the right atmosphere to calm everything down. The parasympathetic system gets bogged down with way too much work because the sympathetic system created all of this tension in our bodies. You see how it works, it's supposed to be a balancing act but the sympathetic "fight or flight" part of our nervous system has created havoc. Our bodies will get hard and create the pain issues mentioned above and our digestion system will begin to have issues as well. The sympathetic system shuts down the digestive system until a later time. Our body's digestive system will not be working very well.

Generally, the harder the muscles the more likely they are to have digestive issues. What might happen soon is people will begin to understand what healthy bodies feel like. The words we use to describe the body will change. People might not say they want to tone up their muscles. Being hard will not be ideal. Both are misleading ideas will soon change as a pliable, rubbery, elastic body will now be seen as the pinnacle of physical and mental health."

In the book I wrote 8 years ago, I came up with a hard body scale. Where soft bodies were a 1 all the way up to 5 who were the hard bodies. I called 3 in between. But in reality, I think our bodies are more a binary machine. Either you are a hard body or a soft body. If you have a way to not hold on to the stress in your life you are a soft body. If you hold onto stress then you are a hard body. There really isn't a halfway.

You learn the most from extremes. I always talk to the soft bodies and find out what they have in common. Then, I do the same with the hard bodies. What do they have in common with other people with hard bodies. After a few years of talking with people this extreme it becomes clear what is going on with their muscles.

Hard Body Issues:

Pain, tingling, numbness, weakness in the arms, hands, legs, or feet.

Headaches

TMJ issues (pain, biting or grinding issues)

Wrist pain (in the carpal tunnel region)

Sciatic pain, numbness
Upper back or neck pain
Shoulder pain

There is also a condition that goes along with this hard body:
You have issues with digestion.

Chapter 8

FASCIA

Fascia is the connective tissue that holds the muscles and organs in place. It is the outer casing of the muscle that also runs throughout the deep layers of the muscles and organs. You can think of it as sausage casing. fascia can get bunched up and cause the muscles to lose some of their length and flexibility. You can feel in get bunched up in some people around the hips, the glutes, and the sides of the upper legs. I work on stretching this superficial layer of spidery webbing. This allows the muscles to regain some length which can help with some structural and pain issues.

Chapter 9

BRIEF DESCRIPTION OF NEUROMUSCULAR

MASSAGE THERAPY AND OTHER MODALITIES

*My bodywork is an integrated or mixed approach
of the following phrases and modalities.*

Body Assessment

All sessions include a body assessment which inform the client which type of body style they have. People have hard or soft muscles that might help explain their pain issues. Also, range of motion (of joints) varies from one person to the next. Tight muscles or specific problem areas can be discussed. Overall body structure or posture influenced by muscles can be examined. Toxins being held in the muscle can be seen visually.

A person's body type will generally influence what kind of massage they like. A soft body can handle quite a bit of pressure because their muscles are healthy, full of blood and oxygen. A hard body will also like a lot of pressure as well, because they can't feel the massage otherwise. A soft body will be able to handle moderate but not too intense work on their tight, hard areas. A hard body will have many trigger points and tight areas that cannot stand much pressure.

People who are holding toxins/fat in their muscles, seen visually, can typically only stand very light work. When a client tells me what kind of pressure they like, I use try to figure out how this corresponds to their body.

Neuromuscular Massage Therapy

NMT is a problem-solving massage style that seeks to release tight areas in a particular muscle. The muscle will concentrate tightness in a specific area rather than creating the tightness throughout. These tight areas are called trigger points. Trigger points can refer pain into the involved muscle or muscles nearby. Trigger points can be seen visually when I work them. I will see a twitching in the area where the trigger point is spreading referred nerve impulse. The client will feel the sensation as a bit of intensity and referred pain or tingling. Hard pressure is not needed to release these trigger points. It is a very subtle medium pressure that is needed to stimulate and get the area to release its tension. I may look at your posture, joint range-of-motion, and treat trigger points and nerve entrapment Neuromuscular Therapy will be used to address five elements that cause pain:

Ischemia: Lack of blood supply to soft tissues which cause hyper-sensitivity to touch.

Trigger Points: Highly irritated points in muscles which refer pain to other parts of the body.

Nerve Compression or Entrapment: Pressure on a nerve by soft tissue, cartilage or bone.

Postural Distortion: Imbalance of the muscular system resulting from the movement of the body off the longitudinal and horizontal planes.

Biomechanical Dysfunction: Imbalance of the musculoskeletal system resulting in faulty movement patterns (i.e., poor lifting habits, bad mechanics in a golf swing of tennis stroke, computer keyboarding.)

Sports Massage

Sports Massage sessions are for those looking for pain relief and restore flexibility. The focus of the massage is to release tight muscles, reduce adhesions and increase range of motion. Also, the fascia of the muscle can be unwound or lengthened. Fascia is the soft tissue component of the connective tissue that provides support and protection for most structures within the human body, including muscle. Fascia can be a superficial layer of muscle that surrounds or encases a muscle. Think of it like a wet suit that keeps the muscle bound in place. Have you ever seen the thin white layer between the skin and the meat of a raw piece of chicken breast? That's fascia. The fascia also runs through the deep layers and medium deep layers of all of the organs and muscles. It holds everything together. This soft tissue can become restricted due to psychogenic disease, overuse, trauma, infectious agents, or inactivity, often resulting in pain, muscle tension, and corresponding diminished blood flow. Although fascia and its corresponding muscle are the main targets of Fascia release, other tissue may be affected as well, including other connective tissue.

Swedish Massage

A Swedish massage can be slow and gentle, or vigorous and stimulating, depending on the therapist's personal style and what he or she wants to achieve. This is not always a superficial massage. It can reach the deep layers. Swedish Massage is characterized by the use of five basic stroke techniques: effleurage, petrissage, friction, tapotement, and vibration.

Chapter 10

CONCLUSION

In conclusion, There are many ways I assess a client on my massage table.

First, I check the overall resting muscle tone of the client's body and determine if I am working on a hard body or soft body. I look for a balanced structure. If it is imbalanced, I try to find if certain muscle groups are tight which are creating the imbalance. I check the range of motion of all of the large muscle groups. I especially check the range of motion where the arms connect to the shoulder and where the legs connect to the hip. I check to see how tight the Iliopsoas muscle is.

I also check for places the fascia needs to be lengthened, especially around the hip joints. I try to soften and relax any areas of tightness the person may be holding in their muscles This is easier to do on a soft body than a hard body. I look for toxins in the muscles. I looked for "bunched up" or restricted fascia. I check for trigger points and tight areas in specific muscles. I talk to clients about their life and lifestyle and try to connect it to their body type.

I look for any structural issues the client has and help the body find a balanced solution. This usually involves lengthening, softening, releasing or unwinding the involved muscles or fascia. It's all about creating space in the muscle. Creating softness where there is denseness, hardness, or shortness.

I'm privileged to take part in this massage revolution that is sweeping the country. It's encouraging to see how massage therapists have the potential of moving health care towards a more preventative and hands-on approach. Let's keep this revolution going.

www.ingramcontent.com/pod-product-compliance
Lightning Source LLC
Chambersburg PA
CBHW060634280326
41933CB00012B/2033